I0103152

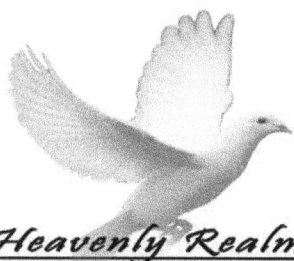

Heavenly Realm Publishing

Houston, Texas

Copyright © 2014 Stephanie Franklin, REshape YOU: *A Fitness Guide to Teach You How to Create the NEW YOU from the Inside Out. All rights reserved.*

Published By: Heavenly Realm Publishing
P. O. Box 682532, Houston, TX 77268
www.heavenlyrealmpublishing.com
Toll Free 1-866-216-0696

Printed in the United States of America

All rights reserved. No part of this book may be reproduced, stored in a retrieval system, or transmitted by any means, electronic, mechanical, photocopying, recording, or otherwise, without written permission from the author.

ISBN—13: 9781937911-87-4 (paperback)
ISBN—13: 9781937911-88-1 (ebook)

Library of Congress Cataloging-in-Publication Data: 2015931410
Stephanie Franklin
REshape YOU: *A Fitness Guide to Teach You How to Create the NEW YOU from the Inside Out/* Stephanie Franklin

1. Health & Fitness: Exercise—United States. 2. Health & Fitness: Healthy Living—United States. 3. Health & Fitness: Healing—United States.

This book is printed on acid free paper.

Scripture quotations are from the Holy Bible. All rights reserved.

Stephanie Franklin
Stephanie Franklin Ministries
PO Box 682532
Houston, TX 77268

REshape YOU

HEART. MIND. BODY. SOUL

*A Fitness Guide to Teach You How to Create the **NEW YOU** from the Inside Out.*

*Achieve Greatness in **YOU**!*

- ✓ Quick Weight Loss
- ✓ Obesity Workouts & Quick Weight Loss
- ✓ Great Exercises, Targeting Your Goal
- ✓ Mental & Emotional Change
- ✓ Family Fitness
- ✓ Inner Healing: HEART* MIND* BODY* SOUL

Bonus: Diabetic Eating Plan & Workout
Personal Eating Plans & Workouts

Stephanie Franklin

Target Areas

- Burn Fat (Arms, legs, calves, thighs, stomach, back, shoulders, etc.)
- Lose Weight
- Right or Better Eating Plans
- Tone Your Muscles
- Learn How to Have Great Health
- How to Gain Weight the Healthy Way
- Better Eating Habits
- Look Great
- Motivation in Yourself
- Feel Great
- Fast Results
- Agility/ Endurance/ Strength Training
- Rehabilitation in Your Body (muscles)
- Body Rehabilitation From Injuries & Surgery
- New Heart
- New Mind
- New Body
- New Soul
- **NEW LOOK!**

RE*shape* YOU

Achieve Greatness in **YOU**!
Create the **NEW YOU** *from the Inside Out!*

Contents:

Chapter One
The Health (HEART) Plan
- ✓ Consider your health.
- ✓ Think about your God given purpose.
- ✓ Put on your Whole Armor
- ✓ Go after it!
- ❖ TAKE THE **HEART** CHALLENGE

Chapter Two
The Mental (MIND) Plan
- ✓ Having a made up mind to consider your health.
- ✓ Being determined to POWER UP mentally
- ✓ You are what you think—*You can if you think you can*
- ✓ Expose the limits in every potential and inabilities
- ✓ Take off the mental limitation barrier
- ✓ Mental to action
- ✓ Don't let the lack of money stop you
- ❖ TAKE THE **MENTAL** CHALLENGE

FICTION NOVELS & MOTIVATIONAL BOOKS:

1. When Ramona Got Her Groove Back from God
2. My Song of Solomon
3. My Song of Solomon *Prayer Journal*
4. God Loves Thugs Too!
5. *The Locker Room Experience: For the Struggling Athlete & Coach, & Tips on How to Get Recruited in Sports*
6. REshape YOU: *A Fitness Guide to Teach You How to Create the NEW YOU from the Inside Out*

MINISTRY BOOKS & WORKBOOK:

7. Position Your Faith for Great Success
8. Position Your Faith for Great Success *Workbook*
9. The Purpose Chaser: *For Children Ages 5 to 12*
10. Church Hurt: *How to Heal & Overcome It*
11. The Power of Healing
12. The Power of the Holy Spirit
13. Winning Together: *His Needs Matter, Her Needs Are Important*
14. Winning Together as a Parent

"Know the <u>power</u> you possess within and use it."

—Stephanie Franklin

REshape YOU

HEART. MIND. BODY. SOUL

Please Be Advised

Although the eating plans and exercises recommended in this book are very simple and harmless, please be advised that each eating plan and exercise may be too rigorous for some. Each level of eating plan and exercise in this book are <u>not</u> intended to hurt, harm, or injure those who try them.

If you feel that they are too rigorous, please consult your physician or those who assist you before beginning.

From the Inside Out

There is a great analogy about *REshape YOU*. *REshape YOU* comes as the Potter and the clay (Jeremiah 18:4-6). God is represented as the Potter, in which shapes and REshapes, molds and REmolds, models and REmodels the clay. The clay, in which is represented as the willing vessel (you and me). The one who <u>allows</u> God to REshape them and do all those things needed to make them into a **totally NEW person.**

I am a firm believer that a person cannot change the outside and stay changed, until the internal them (the inside of them) is completely changed. For example, you can lose weight on the outside; however, if the inside is not changed (bad eating habits, constant junk food eater, speaking negative of yourself and doing the negative of what you speak, no confidence in yourself, low self-esteem, and so on), the weight will come back and most times worse than it was before you lost it in the first place.

Look below at the break down of chain reactions that hinder:

1. <u>Heart</u>- the way you feel about yourself, past hurts, disappointments, guilt, shame of how unattractive you think you look, past mistakes and failures, the hurt and anger of not being

loved, and so hurt and angry that you do not want to receive help from others.

2. **Mind**- thinking less of yourself, feeling unloved within, mental and emotional rejection, laziness and don't know how to come out of it, loss of who you are, thinking you'll never lose the weight, thinking you'll never be able to have healthy eating habits, and suicidal thoughts of giving up with no hope in your future.

3. **Body**- gave up to gluttony (excessive over eating), excessive weight gain, poor eating habits (junk foods, sodas, and fast food takeout's), inconsistent eating habits- eat today but not tomorrow or eat in the morning but not at night, inconsistent workouts, and poor workout plans.

4. **Soul**- Have no spiritual hope for yourself, your faith is withered within, do not believe that you can be REshaped into a NEW person and get a NEW YOU in your life.

REshape YOU was brought about by Stephanie out of concern for the person who not only desire to have better health by taking special care of their body, but also through believing and being healed within one's self; and successful fitness for the entire body. Her goal is to turn all of the negative chain reactions into positive chain reactions that will change one's life forever.

It is God's will that we prosper in health, each day that our souls and bodies prosper (3 John 1:2). It is God's goal that we all take good care of our bodies. What this means is that we are not only striving to be healthy spiritually, but we also strive to exercise and keep our bodies healthy through fitness on a daily and weekly basis. While most of us have not conquered this important goal, I encourage you to start from the beginning and work your way there until it becomes a part of your life. Whatever you do, DO NOT GIVE UP!

Decades after I came out of my teen years of being athletically and physically fit and in the best shape of my life, one day I looked in the mirror and quickly realized that I no longer had that physically fit body like I used too. I had gained over 50 pounds and struggling not only in my body, but also with my self-esteem and faith to look and feel good about myself again. I could literally kill myself because I hated how I looked and wondered if anyone else agreed. I was not used to my bodily flesh growing in places that I had never imagined. And, I don't mean muscles... It also did not help the fact that diabetes run in my family and I did not want to be a victim. This made me realize that I needed to step my game up and eat better, get back in the gym, and get fit. I needed a RE*shaping* from the inside out. I needed a mental, emotional, and physical change. How about you? Are you saying and feeling the same way I did? I encourage you to believe for a RE*shaping* in your life. You'll never be the same.

An important fact I have found to be true through my over 30 year experience in athletics, training, rehabilitation, and coaching, was that many people try many different diet and eating plans, and as they lose weight from the diet or eating plans, their skin sags from the rapid weight loss. This happens as a result of being imbalanced. Being imbalanced come when only one method like dieting and/or training is being used and not both. For example, you cannot work (burn fat) one part of your body in hopes to change it all (lose weight and/or not tone at the same time), you must work (burn fat) all of the body to make it all come together at the same time. Look below to see what I mean:

1. **Dieting-** (successful eating plan for a healthy body).
2. **Weight lifting-** (for muscle tone and/or bodybuilding as you lose the weight your muscles will not sag).
3. **Walking or Running-** (for cardio for the heart and lungs to supply oxygen, and blood to work the muscles in order to work the muscle tissues and use oxygen to produce energy for movement).

Introduction: REshape YOU

There is a balance when it comes to weight loss and looking healthy and great. As you lose weight through a great eating plan, you must also exercise by running, and/or doing aerobics, and/or strength training, and/or agilities, and/or bodybuilding, etc.), and tone your body as the weight decreases—all at the same time. As your weight decreases, sag (the result of a decrease in body fat) will not have a chance to come because you are burning fat <u>and</u> toning as you lose the weight all at the same time. Makes sense? I sure hope so.

As you do these two steps—establish an effective eating plan and workout plan the **NEW REshaped YOU** look is sure to come immediately. There is one last important thing I forgot to mention. The most important thing you need as you go through your daily routine is prayer and believing God for your healing through the reading of His Word. I am a firm Believer that healing comes through your faith to believe you are healed, and by believing God. This part is for your soul and faith, which is needed to believe you can lose and look great in every workout.

Below are the steps that have worked for me, and it can work for you as well:

1. Have confidence in yourself by changing old habits to a lifestyle of better health and fitness on a daily basis, as you BELIEVE for change.

2. Trust God and BELIEVE that you are healed through the reading of His Word about your situation and/or sickness. Find scriptures that target your sickness, health challenge, excessive weight gain, or situation, and joint them down, confess, and study them each day.

3. Research and accomplish a proper exercise and eating plan on a daily basis (establish an effective eating plan and workout plan that works just for you. One only you know you can do each day and excel in it).

REshape YOU has come to help you with each step as it takes you as the reader, the pre-REshape YOU honoree, through every step until you have won in each of these areas to become REshaped.

You have looked at different exercise books, videos, DVD's, and you have almost attempted to try them all yourself. However, as you have tried them all, your strength could not allow you to do them. This is why I have designed this very simple exercise book just for you. I have also included an eating plan and workout plan that will help you as you successfully complete the exercises and use them as a way of life. Each exercise will help you get your blood circulating, not only rapid weight loss, but also with toning and burning excessive fat and carbs.

If you have someone who is able to assist you or a workout partner or even a group, they are encouraged to join in with you. They can help motivate and push you to complete the tasks.

RE*shape* YOU is about doing surgery on your heart (body), mind, spirit, and soul. It goes past just trying to get physically fit, or the popularity of fitness that everyone is seeking. It is about taking what is hindering your progress with progressing to the NEW level that you so desire and need to be on.

- ➤ Are you concerned about your health?
- ➤ Want to learn how to have better eating habits?
- ➤ Want to lose weight overnight?
- ➤ Tone up fast?
- ➤ Learn how to stop procrastinating?
- ➤ Spiritually drained?
- ➤ Body fatigue?
- ➤ Mental & emotional fatigue?
- ➤ Need and want a NEW look?
- ➤ Better health?

RE*shape* YOU will help answer questions and change all of your concerns. Read on...

Items Needed for the RE*shape* YOU Exercises:

1. Faith, mental, motivation, and determination to do whatever it takes to RE*shape* yourself.
2. Chair or bench, bed, couch, track, and/or room floor.
3. Workout mat.
4. Workout gloves *(recommended)*.
5. 8 oz bottle water(s) or cooler with water.
6. Stop watch or a watch with a second hand.
7. T-Shirt or comfortable workout shirt.
8. Walking shorts, warm-ups, or workout tights with shorts.
9. Socks.
10. Exercise athletic shoes *(tennis shoes or walking shoes)*.
11. Towel.
12. Gym bag or workout bag.
13. Dumbbells (hand weights) 2-25lbs. <u>You will need two dumbbells, one for each hand</u>. Use the weight that fits your max weight for a good (max) workout. For example, 2 lbs. or 3 lbs. or 5 lbs. or 8 lbs. or 10 lbs. or 15 lbs. or 20 lbs. or 25 lbs. or higher.

- For **<u>Beginner Level,</u>** weight recommended: 2-3 lbs.
- For **<u>Immediate Level,</u>** weight recommended: 5, 8, 10, or 15 lbs.
- For **<u>Senior Pro Level</u>**, weight recommended: 20-45 lbs. or higher (max weight).

QUICK QUESTIONS TO ANSWER BEFORE YOU BEGIN

Before beginning, please answer the following questions.

Choose Your Workout Level

EXERCISE LEVEL ADD ✓ BELOW	
1. Beginners Level	
2. Immediate Level	
3. Senior Pro Level	

After you have chosen the workout level you are currently on, follow that level throughout the book.

DO YOU CURRENTLY HAVE? *(you may select more than one)*

DIABETES ☐ YES ☐ NO
CANCER ☐ YES ☐ NO
HIGH BLOOD PRESSURE ☐ YES ☐ NO
☐ OTHER, *(please state)* _____
☐ ADDITIONAL MEDICAL HISTORY _____
_____

WHAT ARE YOUR INJURIES? *(only if it applies)*

☐ HEAD
☐ ARM
☐ HAND
☐ KNEE
☐ DO NOT HAVE ANY

☐ ANCLE
☐ WRIST
☐ OTHER, *(please state)* _____
_____

Quick Questions to Answer Before You Begin

WHAT ARE YOUR STRENTGHS? *(you may select more than one)*

☐ UPPER BODY:
arms ___ chest___ stomach ___ all___

☐ LOWER BODY:
Legs: thighs ___ calves ___ ankles ___ all ___

☐ RUNNING
☐ WALKING
☐ HIKING
☐ SWIMMING
☐ WEIGHT LIFTING
☐ RACE WALKING *(fast pace walk)*

☐ AROBICS
☐ CHEST
☐ STOMACH
☐ SIT-UPS
☐ PUSH-UPS
☐ BICYCLING
☐ OTHER, *(please state)* _____
_____

WHAT ARE YOUR WEAKNESSES? *(you may select more than one)*

☐ UPPER BODY:
arms ___ chest___ stomach ___ all___

☐ LOWER BODY:
Legs: thighs ___ calves ___ ankles ___ all ___

☐ EATING CANDY
☐ SOFT DRINKS
☐ RUNNING
☐ SLOW WALKING
☐ HIKING
☐ AROBICS
☐ SIT-UPS
☐ PUSH-UPS
☐ SWIMMING

☐ SITTING, WATCHING TV
☐ CHEST
☐ DO NOT TAKE VITAMINS
☐ DO NOT TAKE VITAMINS
REGULARLY
☐ RACE WALKING *(fast pace walk)*
☐ WEIGHT LIFTING
☐ BICYCLING
☐ HIKING
☐ AROBICS
☐ OTHER, *(please state)* _____
_____

WHAT ARE YOUR TARGET AREAS? *(you may select more than one)*

☐ BURN FAT
☐ MUSCLE INCREASE
☐ LOSE WEIGHT
☐ GAIN WEIGHT
☐ INCREASE POWER
☐ LOSE STOMACH
☐ BODY BUILDING MAXING

☐ INCREASE FOOT WORK *(agility)*
☐ INCREASE SPEED
☐ INCREASE ENDURANCE
☐ INCREASE UPPER BODY STRENTGH
☐ OTHER, *(please state)* _____
_____

WEIGH IN CHART & DOCUMENTATION *(do not weigh before due date)*

WHAT YOU WEIGH NOW:	DATE:
WEEK 1	DATE:
WEEK 5	DATE:
WEEK 8	DATE:
WEEK 12	DATE:

23

Stephanie Franklin

Start Weigh Chart Over After your Week 12:	
WEEK 1:	DATE:
WEEK 5:	DATE:
WEEK 8:	DATE:
WEEK 12:	DATE:

YOUR FITNESS GOAL *(write your goal(s) below)*

_____
_____
_____
_____
_____
_____

YOUR HEALTH GOAL *(write your goal(s) below)*

_____
_____
_____
_____
_____
_____

Quick Questions to Answer Before You Begin

| PHOTO GOES BELOW: *(take before you begin)* | |
BEFORE	AFTER 8 or 12-WEEKS

MY DAILY EATING PLAN CHART:

- MONDAY
- TUESDAY
- WEDNESDAY
- THURSDAY
- FRIDAY
- SATURDAY
- SUNDAY

Stephanie Franklin

Now that you have completed the questions and have taken your before photo and have pasted it on the before photo area, you are ready to begin. If you have not taken your photo or choose not to, you can still begin now.

Ready? LET'S GET STARTED...

Chapter One

The Health (HEART) Plan

In thinking of "the Health (HEART) Plan", one would think in terms of:

- ✓ Consider your health.
- ✓ Think about your God-given purpose.
- ✓ Put on your Whole Armor *(your complete workout gear)*, ready to get started.
- ✓ Go after it!

❖ **TAKE THE HEART CHALLENGE**

The Health (HEART) Plan

✓ **Consider your health.**

It is important to have a plan in place for everything you need in order to have a successful life each day of your life. In this case, I am speaking of the heart. It is important to consider your health at all times and at all cost. Many people are lacking in the area of keeping their heart healthy by the lifestyles they live.

Although there are some heart diseases that are beyond our control, below are types of areas that hinder the heart from functioning correctly and may bring heart disease:

1. Smoking. Nicotine inhalation can produce a heart attack.
2. Gluttony. Obesity (Constantly over eating).
3. Bad Eating Habits (lack vitamins and healthy foods).
4. Alcoholic. Drinking too much can bring heart attacks, high blood pressure, obesity, stroke, breast cancer.
5. Lack of proper exercise.

These types of points can bring sickness, which weighs on the heart. If the heart does not function properly, it will shut down, leave the person paralyzed, without the ability to speak or get around physically, or even deceased. It was never ordained for the heart to have an extreme amount of pressure on it. It is ordained to be peaceful and relaxed and pumping healthy. This is how it continues to beat strongly each day.

Fear is a hindrance when it comes to having a healthy heart. Fear stirs up all sorts of emotions and enzymes within the body. Enzymes are biological molecules *(proteins)* that significantly speed up the rate of virtually all the chemical reactions that take place within cells in your body. They are vital for life and serve a wide range of functions within the body. They aide metabolism and digestion.

Fear brings sickness and stress on your body. It puts pressure on your heart. It affects your thinking and your heart rate increases. If you are experiencing fear and sicknesses, below are some helpful tips that will help you to overcome them.

THE HELPFUL TIP:

1. Do not accept fear. Tell yourself, "I do not accept fear".
2. Stop smoking.
3. Watch your eating intake.
4. Watch what you eat.
5. Be alcohol free.
6. Get plenty of exercise.
7. Drink plenty of water.
8. Make annual doctor visits. There is nothing wrong with annual check-ups.

In order to rid these sicknesses, know that it is not only in getting plenty of exercise, it is also mostly important to change the way you think. Are you thinking negative about yourself? If so, Why?

_____

_____

Are you trying to change from this negative way of thinking? _____Why or Why not? _____

_____.

This way of thinking occurs in the mind. You must change what you allow to sit on your mind. If you <u>think</u> you cannot accomplish something, then you will not. If you <u>think</u> you cannot lose weight, then you will not. If you <u>think</u> you cannot have great eating habits, then you will not. Your faith must line up with your physical will. You must say, "I have a will to workout 5 days a week and I am going to lose 50 pounds in 4 weeks." This is <u>thinking</u> faith. You can actually believe that you have already lost the weight. When you think like this, it will come faster and you will feel great!

✓ **Think about your God-given purpose.**

Think about your God-given purpose. When you think about your God-given purpose, your health should come to mind. It would be very hard to fulfill your God-given purpose when you are not healthy. It is hard to live day by day when you are sick in your body. You have to make up in your mind that you are going to take charge of your health and not allow the pressures of life and negative eating habits to pull you down to a life of defeat. Set a goal that today you are going to follow the Helpful Tip above and win in those areas everyday of your life.

A healthy mind is the result of a healthy body. If you are sick, there is no way you can think straight. All you are thinking about is the sickness you have, while praying it'll go away. You are literally bound to that sickness while nothing gets accomplished. However, when you are healthy and feeling great, your mind is free and able to think properly as you accomplish your God-given purpose. Fitness and a proper eating plan play a huge role in you completing your God-given purpose. Consider it today.

✓ **Put on your Whole Armor** *(your complete workout gear)*, **ready to get started.**

Bring your Whole Armour (Your complete workout gear), ready to start. You should always be prepared. You should never let anyone catch you slipping and unprepared.

The Whole Armour derives from the Bible (Ephesians 6:11-18) as being a complete full covering ready for war, and not allowing anything and anyone to penetrate through to harm or hinder you from head to toe from receiving your best. It is also your gear to war against the fight of setback and excessive body fat that is trying to overtake you. This is the same thing when it comes to protecting your health and your heart. You should cover yourself in such a way that bad habits, negative lifestyles, and negative people will not be able to come in, penetrate through your Armour, and hurt you. While none of us is perfect, you should strive for perfection each day, and do your best to follow the plan that is set before you and make a goal to complete it.

Tom arrived right on time to fitness class. He decided to change up. He wore his steel toe boots to class instead of his athletic shoes that he always wears. He realized after looking in his gym bag that he'd forgotten his athletic shoes. "I can't believe I left my shoes." He exclaimed as Jeff, his workout partner heard him and asked.

"What's going on Tom? Ready to workout?"

"Unfortunately I'm not. I left my athletic shoes and there's no way I can workout in these steel toe boots."

Jeff looked him up and down and said. "Wow the boots huh'? Not your normal workout gear. I hate that you're not fully prepared. I looked forward to working out with you today."

"Yea', well, unfortunately I'm ganna' have to take a rain check. I gotta' go home today. Home's too far for me to go and come back."

The question is, was Tom fully geared up? Did he come prepared like he always do? Do not take chances on changing your routine of doing things right. If the same fully prepared way is working for you, why fix it or change it? Has this ever been you? Remember, it pays to come prepared and covered so that you can get what you need.

Joan has been trying so hard to make a change in her bad eating habits and trying to lose her obesity weight that the doctor warned her to lose. She is trying so hard to stay determined as she prepares to leave home to go to strength training. "John, I'm on my way to strength training. Be back later!" She yelled waiting for a response.

John yells from the other room. "I don't know why you're going, it ain't ganna' help you any!"

Joan immediately stops in her tracks, sits down at the kitchen table, and begins to cry. She has lost her determination and drive to keep going.

It is important to cover yourself and not allow negative feedback to make you lose your determination and momentum to make a change for yourself. Let your Whole Armour cover you as you go forth to win in negative situations like that one with John. Turn it around with a positive gestor and keep it moving, let negativity know that it or those person(s) will not get the best of you, and work harder to show that you will not quit but let it make you stronger to win against all odds.

✓ **Go after it!**
Go after it! Your new life and new plan is before you. Let's Go!

TAKE THE HEART CHALLENGE

Challenge #1
Learn the heart you have. Dissect areas within your heart that
may be affecting your health and exercise progress. (EX: stress,
anger, fear, worry).

Challenge #2
Know your risks of heart disease. Get a check-up/physical
annually.

Challenge #3
Begin exercising with a challenging workout plan and a
workable eating plan fit just for you.

Chapter Two

The Mental (MIND) Plan

In thinking of "the Mental (MIND) Plan", one would think in terms of:

- ✓ Having a made up mind to consider your health.
- ✓ Being determined to POWER UP mentally
- ✓ You are what you think—*You can if you think you can*
- ✓ Expose the limits in every potential and inability
- ✓ Take off the mental limitation barrier
- ✓ Mental to action
- ✓ Don't let the lack of money stop you
- ❖ **TAKE THE MENTAL CHALLENGE**

The Mental (MIND) Plan

We've all heard this powerful saying, "a mind is a terrible thing to waste". Well, I say when the mind is wasted, the entire body is wasted. There is absolutely nothing you can do with your body when your mind is not functioning properly. The mind will make you do all sorts of things you have never dreamed of doing. This is why it is so important to protect your mind with positive,

35

winning thoughts—thoughts to win over what is negatively nagging you to lose.

When your thoughts are on positive things, it will be easy to say, think, and do positive things. When your mind is always thinking negative, it will make you say, think, and do negative things. The problem with thinking negative is, you'll always repeat these things until you release the cycle and choose to turn your thoughts into positive, winning thoughts.

You may ask, "how do I release the cycle?" I will answer:

1. Ask God for positive thoughts daily.
2. Watch what you speak and how you speak.
3. Watch what you think.
4. Watch what you do.
5. Watch what you allow to embed in your mind.
6. Change your mentality from negative defeat, to positive victory—you win not lose mindset.
7. Walk in the mentally REshaped YOU attitude daily.

It is important to have a mental health plan in place. Your mental health plan should include nothing but a faith, winning plan. It should not look like the defeated mentality of where you may have come from, but it should look like the determined attitude of, you will win and overcome the obstacles that have kept you down from where you are going. If you have gained weight and

The Mental (MIND) Plan

feel as if there is no possible way you can lose the weight, this is a defeated mental attitude. I used to have this mentality. And I lost every time. Pounds never shed. But the minute I made up in my mind and established a mental health plan, I began to win. I quickly researched myself to find out what I was doing wrong, and what was keeping me from losing the weight. I quickly found out that it was not the fact that I was not working out or eating right at the moment, the root of it was the negative way I thought and spoke about myself. Therefore, I had to change the way I spoke and thought in terms of being confident in losing the weight and being successful in eating right. When you do not have confidence in yourself and what you are capable of doing will keep you from your best.

You are depriving yourself from your greatest potential. Millions of people across the globe are losing in this area. They are settling for less than what they can be for fear of trying and thinking they will lose in their trying. This is not always that case. You will never know until you try. God does not make junk. He is always waiting to help you when you step out on faith, take a stand, and try.

You must cast down imaginations that will make you think in a way that your current situation will not get better, as your thoughts overcome you with evil thoughts and emotions of defeat. You must change those thoughts into thoughts of, "I will win no matter what because I am not a failure." "I will win no matter what I feel like at this moment." "I will workout no matter what my mind is telling me, I can and will accomplish it today." "I will lose weight and eat better today. I'm on my way and I feel great!" "I will overcome setbacks in my life that constantly tell me to quit and to give up." This is what you literally have to say to yourself everyday until you are, and feel confident within yourself.

If heavy weight is the issue and you feel as though it cannot change or you will never get the size or the physical fit that you so desire, you must change those thoughts because those are thoughts of defeat and you are lowering your greatest potential to create the NEW REshaped YOU. We have seen it on television and we have read it in newspapers, magazines, and books about how many have REshaped themselves from the old look to the NEW look from the inside out. You are no different, since they did it, you can do it too. Do you believe that? I certainly do.

✓ **Having a made up mind to consider your health.**
Having a made up mind to consider your health is a mind that refuse to stay in its current let down (the woe it's me attitude and pity party), defeated, setback, or blaming others for your failures situation any longer. This is when you refuse to have a sick mentality, sick mind, or a body wearied down with infirmity.

This means you are going to do whatever it takes to get your body healthy and keep it healthy. Do you agree? I believe so.

An effective, rigorous daily workout and eating plan helps in this area. One that is just right for you, that is. Also, annual flushing of your body's toxic is also good. This will steer you in the right direction to remove all of those setbacks that I have mentioned above.

✓ **Being determined to POWER UP mentally**

To POWER UP mentally is to immediately get yourself pumped up and ready to REshape YOU from the inside out. What this means is that you are getting yourself ready for the NEW level, NEW faith, and NEW journey to your NEW life of a NEW person, NEW positive determined outlook, and NEW faith and NEW power to believe to move forward and not to turn back. Ask yourself, "Am I ready to POWER UP?" You can answer that question all by yourself. "I am ready the POWER UP, and I am determined!"

Ever watched a motivational movie or program, or went to see an exciting sporting event, and afterwards you were so motivated that you believed that you could conquer the world? You were ready to face anything that came your way? You could run a 10 K marathon in a flash? You could go out and lift all the weights in the gym that day? Well, I want you to know that your faith and motivation to win and to POWER UP was just that high that it caused you to change from your current everyday o' well attitude, to an immediate supernatural up-lifted change into a NEW REshape YOU person you were designed and meant to be. This is the person and POWER UP attitude I am speaking of. If the greatest athletes or people you know who are in tip-top shape can do it and win, so can you. POWER UP!

I tell my personal trainees and boot camp groups that I personally train to POWER UP! I encourage them to FAITH UP as well! Stir your faith up to believe that you can do the impossible and believe in yourself, no matter what you look like and your current situation looks like right now. Believe that you and it will not stay that way always, you will come out of it, and you will make an immediate change from the inside out by faith. My personal training and boot camp program teaches this and it has worked successfully with youth, men and women giving success stories like, "Since I tried Ms. Stephanie's personal training and boot camp program, I have never been the same—mentally, emotionally, athletically, physically (weight wise), and I have a new faith—I'm different in the way that I look at things and life. I believe in myself now. I feel great and I don't feel tired and want to give up. I want to workout and I now know that I look great since I lost the weight!" Here's one more, "I am no longer the same, my bad habits have changed. I don't think the way I used to think—defeated and don't care."

Have a NEW determination and a NEW mind. I encourage you to POWER UP!

✓ **You are what you think—***You can if you think you can*
There was a mid-aged man who came up to me as I was working out at a gym one day. He struck up a conversation first about how bad he looks and all the blubber he has on his body, as every word that came out of his mouth was negative. There was nothing about his conversation that was positive. In fact, he literally drained me while listening to him. He kept talking, while looking at me as if to taunt me to voice my negative opinions as well. Well, it worked. I began to be negative right along with him. His negative thinking and speaking transferred on me. My positive attitude about working out and bettering myself changed into a defeated headache. Have you ever had this happen to you? Did their mission of transferring negativity with a big ball of self-pity work on you?

A negative thinking person will always expose him or herself as a very negative person. They cannot hide. They will always come out. They are a very unhappy person. They are very unhappy about their life. They are very unhappy about how they look. They are very unhappy about who God made them. They are very unhappy about their negative current situation they are in. They are very unhappy to see others happy. They are very unhappy about how over weight they are. And, most times these types of people want everybody else unhappy right along with them. If one of these are you, it is time to REshape your negative thinking to positive thinking.

As with the mid-aged man, normally I am very positive as doubt and negativity cringes me. I wanted to tell the man if he'd stop being so negative about how he look, about who God made him, and about everything, he would find that it is not as bad as he thinks. You are what you think. If you think you are ugly, then you are ugly. If you think you are fat and will always be, then you will be fat and will always be. If you think you are sick, then you are sick. If you think you have a headache, then you have a headache. If you think you are too out of shape to get in shape and eat better, then you will always be out of shape and have terrible eating habits. If you think you are a loser, then you are a loser. No one can change this negative mentality but you. And, if you choose not to change it, you will find that those around you will become few to none. No one wants to be around a negative person who thinks negative about themselves, about everything, and about everybody all the time. Now-a-days, people are looking for someone who is positive, who can be motivated just as they are, who will motivate them without passing judgment, who wants to live a better life, who wants to look better, feel better, and reach every goal they can get their hands on each day of their lives. Those are the winning people. Those are the POWER UP people. Those are the people who do not think defeated, but think to win. Those are the NEW REshape YOU people.

This is the way you should to be if you are struggling in those negative areas. No one is perfect, however, if you are in error of those areas, have a made up mind to change and turn around every negative, defeated, don't care, jealous, hateful, mean, angry, fearful, and intimidated attitude and mentality you have today. It works. Some of that used to be me. I hope you can find others who were that same way who changed.

✓ **Expose the limits in every potential and inability**
There are millions who are not using the potentials they were born with. They do not use them for either fear, comfortable in their daily lifestyles; have no reason to, and so much more. You have got to expose those areas that you are not exposing your best potential in. It is God's will that you walk in your best everyday and use those gifts and potentials everyday. If they are not used, they become stifled until you no longer are able to operate or fulfill them. You are what you think and you have the opportunity to set a goal and accomplish it. Don't let limitations

hold you back from accomplishing what you set your mind too, use your faith and determination and a positive mindset to set out to do it and do it right until you complete it! Do not quit and do not stop until you complete it. I encourage you!

✓ **Take off the mental limitation barrier**
Take off the limitation barrier of what others say about you. You may have been told that you cannot accomplish anything. You may have been told that you are nothing and will never be anything. You may be suffering from a generational curse of failure and setback. Someone may have attacked your integrity and made you feel less of a person. You may have been told that you are fat and you will always be fat because it runs in your family. You may have also been abused and rejected, and never encouraged to know that you are somebody; and that you can do anything you set your mind to. Therefore, you have made up in your mind and have lived a life to receive these words, actions, or situations that have happened to you. All of these real life examples have come to bring you mental limitation barriers. They have come to set you back from being confident in knowing who you are. They have come to destroy the potential you possess inside to become somebody great. If you have operated in this mentality, either all of your life, or since yesterday, I encourage you to take off the mental limitation barriers.

The Mental (MIND) Plan

Make a choice today that you will not limit yourself any longer by the negative real life examples I just shared of what others have said to you, either in your past or presently. Remove the barriers from your thoughts, mind, and heart and choose to make an immediate turn around today. You will no longer hold up your barriers to keep others out. And, you will no longer push barriers at other people to keep them from loving you, helping you, and encouraging you. You can change, and this is your day to do so if you want it.

✓ **Mental to action**

Go from just thinking that you can, to putting it into action that you can. Go from thinking that it would be nice if you could, to making it nice that you did. Put your thoughts into action. Make your thoughts a reality. You may ask how do I put my thoughts into action? I will answer:

1. Stop procrastinating. You already have the thought that you want to do it. That is the first step. Now all you have to do is stop holding yourself back and get started.

2. Write your goal(s) down. If it's to change the way you eat. Do research and write down a new eating plan—what vegetables to eat, healthy drinks to drink without sugar added that still taste good to

45

you, how to bake your meats without frying them, and how to put your healthy meals together. If it's to challenge yourself to a more rigorous workout to lose weight or tone up your body, then write a new workout plan down. Do research on some rigorous workouts that others are doing and set a goal for yourself and your body and complete them. The internet is full of them. You can also get you a personal trainer and a dietitian (or dietician), who can help you outline those target areas. A dietitian is someone who can advise you on what to eat in order to lead a healthy lifestyle and achieve a specific health-related goal.

3. Go After it! POWER UP! Get out and do it without thinking twice about it. I have learned that once you do it, you feel great and you'll be glad you did. You will also not want to stop when you begin to see fast results.

✓ **Don't let the lack of money stop you**
I challenge you not to let the lack of money stop you from signing up to a great fitness facility, or getting a personal trainer to get a great workout, or finding a great dietitian to help you learn how to eat healthy. It is true that living healthy comes with a higher

The Mental (MIND) Plan

price. Most healthy products cost a little more than normal fatty food products. Although there are some that are cheaper. I believe that when you think about your health and how important it is to live healthy, you will sacrifice the extra money you use to buy unnecessary things. You will be able to use that money to buy healthy products, sign up to a fitness facility or personal trainer, and be able to fund the cost to get fit the way you want to and need to.

Do not be discouraged. If money is still an issue regardless of what I just mentioned, there are many local parks and gyms you can find to go and exercise at that are free. You can do your research and find an eating plan fit just for you (you can try the one in this book) and start with that plan until you can afford to make the investment of the fitness membership or personal trainer or dietitian to fit within your budget.

On the next page, I challenge you to take the mental challenge and apply it to your life and workout on a daily basis.

TAKE THE MENTAL CHALLENGE

Challenge #1
Set a goal to complete this checklist successfully.

- ✓ Having a made up mind to consider your health.
- ✓ Being determined to POWER UP mentally
- ✓ You are what you think—*You can if you think you can*
- ✓ Expose the limits in every potential and inability
- ✓ Take off the mental limitation barrier
- ✓ Mental to action
- ✓ Don't let the lack of money stop you

Challenge #2
Expose the limits in your life that is keeping back your potential(s). Tell yourself, "I will not hide and look from behind my negative past, my hidden talents, and my drive to better me anymore."

Challenge #3
Take off the limitation barriers. Do not allow people to tell you what you can and cannot accomplish. Be confident in your God-given talent and ability to change from the old you into a NEW REshaped YOU.

Challenge #4
Take the limits off. Take the limitation barriers off of, "I can't, it won't happen, that's not for me, that is impossible, or who cares. **REshape** your mind and begin exercising with a challenging workout plan and a workable eating plan that works just for you.

Chapter **Three**

Family—Fit—Together

In thinking of "Family—Fit—Together", one would think in terms of:

- ✓ Family
- ✓ Fit
- ✓ Together
- ❖ **TAKE THE FAMILY WORKOUT CHALLENGE**

Family—Fit—Together

It's time for the family to come together and get fit together! This chapter gets the entire family active and moving—together.

Children and teens spend an awful lot of time watching TV, on their cell phones, on the internet, on social media, and not enough time concentrating on being healthy.

✓ Family

It is important that the family spend time together. I share in my book, "Winning Together: *His Needs Matter, Her Needs Are*

Important" and also in my book, *"Winning Together as a Parent".* Each book gives detailed information on how to win in relationships, as a married couple, and as a family. The reason why I mentioned these books is because I want you to understand how important it is for the married couple (if married) and family as a whole to spend time together as much as possible. In this case, exercise is the key to having a fit family that strives to look and feel healthy as much as possible.

You may ask, "what can the married couple or family do together to get in perfect fit?" I will answer, there are many, however, you only want to choose the ones that are fun and fit for the entire family. Below are some examples I'll give you for married couples and family fitness:

1. Go biking together. You and your spouse or family can ride bikes around the neighborhood or at a local park. What a great way to come together and spend time together while getting a good exercise in for each married couple and for each person in the family. Also for those in a relationship if you're not married.

2. Play the game of tennis together. Play tennis together at a local park or school. What a great way to exercise together and play singles or doubles or just have as many as you want on a

team. The goal is to come together and be together. Also for the married couple if you're married.

3. Go swimming together. You all can go swimming at a local community swimming pool or at home. This is a great way to come together and get great exercise while being together. Also for the married couple if you're married.

4. Do yard work together. Come together and clean the yard, pick up sticks, mow the grass, plant new flowers, etc. This is a great way to come together and exercise and have fun doing it—together. Also for the married couple if you're married.

5. Go mountain climbing. There are now available some of these fun exercises at some of the local fitness centers. You just have to find one. They bring a sense of working together, fun fitness, and appreciation for one another.

Most kids and teens do not like to do exercises that are not hands on or are not on their level. They get bored and choose to stay home while you and your spouse, if any, go alone. I have educated children and youth, and have worked with kids and teens for decades and they all say the same thing, *"I don't want to do nothin' boring."* They want to do things that are fun, as it gives them a good workout. The points I stated are great for your family to take advantage of while it makes each of you stronger and your family bond stronger.

You may say, "I'm a single parent and it is only me and my teen son or daughter. Do I need a huge family in order to get a great workout together?" I will say, no you do not. You do not have to have a huge family in order to get a good workout. A good workout with your family does not come in large sizes, it comes with you working with the family that you have and having fun doing it. And, you do not have to be in tip-top shape to do the exercises above.

Family fit (fitness) helps the family work through the most stressful times, draw closer together, and the parents help groom the children or teen and lead them in the direction they should go. Your children may be adults. It does not matter. You all can enjoy your time together just as if they weren't. This is what makes the family grow stronger. This should be the goal of every family.

✓ Fit
We all know to be healthy and in bodily fit is not only one of the most important things we need in this world, but it is also one of the best feelings that you can have when you are in the best

shape of your life. The average person does not obtain this type of fit (fitness). This is something that they all wish or dream of. *REshape YOU* comes to change all of that. You must have a passion for fitness in order to get in tiptop physical fit. If the passion and the drive is not there, it will be a very hard challenge for you to start, and after you start, it will be very hard to continue.

You must love yourself. Fit (fitness) comes with taking pride in your body no matter how it looks. It may not be an award winning looking body as of yet, but you do not see it in the shape it currently is in, you see it in the shape of the award winning looking body you want it to be. Make sense? Good.

You must have the right mind and attitude in order to experience the fit body you want. It does not work only depending and looking at the outer appearance, it works altogether. Also, do not look at how some else's body looks who has a size 4 shape. Although looking at others who have already accomplished the goal you are looking the accomplish is good, if you are not in a position where it does not bother you or set you back from achieving the fit you need and want, then do not waste your time looking. Everybody's body structure is different. God made you just the way you are. You strive to look and feel great according to the body-fit you have, and not from what someone else's body-fit has. Theirs may be quite different and the results may not turn out the same.

Keeping your body in perfect health plays a huge part in getting the fit body you are looking for.

1. Eat and drink healthy each day. Drink abundance of water, take your vitamins daily, and drink healthy drinks (healthy juicers, protein shakes, etc.).

2. Exercise—pump iron, dance aerobics, strength training, walking, running, or biking.

3. Repeat your performance with the POWER UP attitude each day, each week, and each month of your life.

I encourage you to challenge yourself to reach for the best-fit body you can.

✓ Together

It is important to be together as a family. Family time together allows room for growth, instills more respect, and brings a greater since of closeness.

Just as I mentioned about setting aside family time to workout together, it carries on to this topic. As you as a family have chosen a fun activity to do, make sure that it is together and not what one person wants to do. It is not a selfish thing, it is a together thing. You all make the choice of what fun workout you all would like to do, while making sure it is light and not too hard and too aggressive for your children (if any).

As you show unity within your fun fitness activity, other's watching will be encouraged to do the same. This is why it is important to work together, if married, the husband and wife should make sure to choose family fitness activities that not only fit themselves, but they also fit children and teen-like activities.

If you are already doing this, well done. But there are still many others that are not. I encourage you to do activities that you can do. Be creative as you do these consistently and make them apart of your daily life style—together. These not only are great for memories, but they are good for your health.

TAKE THE FAMILY WORKOUT CHALLENGE

Challenge #1
Challenge yourself to go beyond your comfort zone. Dissect areas within your life that is keeping you from getting together with your family to exercise. You may base it from my personal training workouts or from your own.

Challenge #2
Be persistent and consistent. Show love toward one another as you get a great workout and have fun while doing it.

Challenge #3
Don't quit.

Challenge #4
Take the limits off. Take the limitation barriers off of, "I can't, it won't happen, that's not for me, that is impossible, or who cares." **REshape** your mind and begin exercising with your family and with a challenging workout plan and a workable eating plan that works just for you and your family.

Chapter Four

The Workout (BODY) Plan

In thinking of "the Workout (BODY) Plan", one would think in terms of:

- ✓ Eating plan
- ✓ Stretching
- ✓ Walking
- ✓ Running
- ✓ Obesity workout & quick weight loss eating plan
- ❖ **TAKE THE WORKOUT (BODY) CHALLENGE**

The Workout (BODY) Plan

While everybody's body is different, you have to find a workout plan that works best for your body to receive. You cannot go by what others are doing. However, you can be encouraged by what they are doing and pan you an eating plan and/or workout that fits where <u>you are</u> as you start where you are. Like they say, *"don't try to keep up with the Joneses"*. It will not work because you are not where they are, yet, and you can have potential injuries and setbacks when you go too fast and try to be something, someone, or on a level that you are not yet. For example, trying to bench press 250 pounds because you watched your friend do it, when you have never benched pressed that amount of weight a day in your life. Or, here's another example, you seen someone's eating plan on television and it works for them, so you try that same eating plan which you have never done in your life and it is way too much required and overwhelming, and you get sick. It is nothing wrong with taking some ideas of what others have while taking away and adding to the workout and eating plan to fit your body and lifestyle. This will help you to be able to start and stick with it.

Start where you are and work from there. If you work hard and do not give up, it will not take long and you will pass the Joneses and be well on your way to the NEW REshaped YOU.

✓ **Eating Plan**

Breaking old habits are always hard. Developing a successful eating plan to fit only you is the plan that I shoot for in this chapter. While there are many plans and diet supplements, there is only one plan that can only cater to YOUR specific need. This chapter shoots for that goal to cater to your body, mental, emotional, and spiritual need. Below is one of my many eating plans and workout programs I share to help you balance your workout (the outer), and your daily eating plan (the inner), along with the spiritual (the inner, mental, soul). You may choose to partner up or in a group. It can also be done individually.

✓ Stretching

I teach this to those who I train that stretching is the most important part of the workout before beginning. Stretching is what warms up your muscles and gets them going. It stretches and loosens them up before a hard rigorous workout. When a person does not stretch properly before working out, they have the potential of straining and/or pulling a muscle. Your muscles are very sensitive when it comes to using them, they want to give you what you so desire. So, you have to give them what they desire also and that is preparing them before they are used in order to get what you need.

When the weather is cold, it is important to stretch much more until your muscles are completely stretched and warmed up. A quick jog is also good before and after you stretch as you go into and come out of your workout. Remember, do not abuse your body by thinking that you can get away with not stretching, because it may not always last, especially when you are first starting out and have not workout in a very long time. Most times, you can't feel it right away (during your workout) until you get home and your muscles relax and that's when the soreness, stiffness, and the pain hits you all at once. This is what I am talking about. It is important not to only stretch before you workout and lift weights, but it is also important to workout afterwards.

I used to tell my athletes that I have coached in the past, and those I now train that, you can never stretch enough. But even in your stretching, you want to watch the way you stretch. If you feel your muscles are stretched too much, you want to lower your count. If your muscles are tight and stiff, you want to increase to a higher count to loosen them before walking, running, weight lifting, and/or before any kind of strength training and agility workout.

With my experience in being an athlete, a coach, and a personal trainer, most of them say the same thing, "I don't like to stretch." I have found that most injuries occur from the lack of proper stretching. They can also occur from the lack of a proper workout—either not enough and/or from overdoing it—fatigue.

✓ **Walking**

Walking works hand in hand with a healthy diet/eating plan. It is essential to helping burn fat and getting the lean body you desire. While some people do not want a lean body, they just want to lose the current heavy weight enough for good health and enough to look good in their clothes. Whichever is your choice.

The Workout (BODY) Plan

However, whatever you desire, make sure you target your walking to get max results for a good workout. Do not waste your time. Make the best out of your walking to feel like you have gotten a great workout, rather than the feeling of when you are done to feel like you've just casually walked around your house. It should entail much more than that unless circumstances do not allow.

There are different types of walking you can do, depending on the level you are on. In the beginning of the book, you should have chosen the level you are: the Beginners, the Immediate, or the Senior Pro Level. I coach and train those who are all three of these.

1. For the Beginners Level, your walk should be slow and at a constant pace.

2. For the Immediate Level, you should walk at a consistent medium to fast pace (a race walk pace).

3. For the Senior Pro Level, this is the level for the person who has been working out for a very long time—they are seasoned and are in tiptop shape. Your walk should be a constant fast pace walk on into a running pace. Most use this fast pace walk for a warm up and then afterwards run for best results.

✓ **Running**

Running is a much higher step from walking. It requires a greater expectation than just walking. Running is important for those athletes who are training to get in shape for an event and/or just running to get in shape, better shape, or in tiptop shape.

As you run, you want to make sure that you choose the type of running workout you want to do—a slow, fast, or a sprint run. Whichever is chosen, make sure that you run your max pace for fast and best results. The longer and harder you run, the more fat and calories you burn, and the more weight you lose.

Are you ready to begin the RE*shaping* of your life? Now I must admit, it will be challenging, however, you can do it and I guarantee you, you will never be the same again. Your happy days will come, just do not give up!

Take the workout (body) challenge on the next page before you begin...

TAKE THE WORKOUT (BODY) CHALLENGE

Challenge #1
Challenge yourself to go beyond your comfort zone. Dissect areas within your heart that may be affecting your health and exercise progress. (EX: stress, anger, fear, worry). Make yourself a workout chart that fits your maximum workout strength. You may base it from my personal training workouts or from your own.

Challenge #2
Be persistent and consistent in every workout. Do not be on one day and off the other day(s).

Challenge #3
Don't quit.

Challenge #4
Take the limits off. Take the limitation barriers off of, "I can't, it won't happen, that's not for me, that is impossible, or who cares." **REshape** your mind and begin exercising with a challenging workout plan and a workable eating plan that works just for you.

ENTER THE DATE YOU ARE STARTING THE EATING & WORKOUT PLAN PROGRAM?
_____

ENTER THE DATE YOU ENDED THE EATING & WORKOUT PLAN PROGRAM?
_____

WHAT LEVEL ARE YOU ON? *(LOOK IN FRONT OF BOOK)*
_____

NOW ARE YOU READY? LET'S GET STARTED!

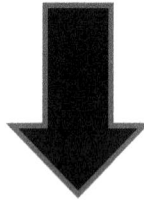

EATING PLAN #1
GOAL: ½ *GALLON OF WATER DAILY*
8 WEEK PROGRAM

********USE THIS EATING PLAN FOR QUICK
WEIGHT LOSS ONLY- FOR 8 WEEKS********

MORNING

1. (1) EGG
2. (1) SLICE OF TOAST
3. 1/2 cup of oatmeal
4. (1) juicer/natural fruit drink and/or protein shake. Drink one in the morning, or noon, or night.
5. (2) 16 oz bottles or cups of water *(must be completed by noon, before lunch)*

NOON

1. (1/2) Sandwich *(wheat bread only)*
2. (1) bag of chips preferably "All Natural Chips or Tortilla Chips"*(no salt)* **-OR-** you may do (1/2 cup) of vegetables in the place of chips.
3. (1/2 cup) of fruit. *Preferably grapes or orange.*
4. (3) 16 oz bottles or cups of water *(must be completed before dinner)*

NIGHT

1. (1 slice) Baked chicken or turkey
2. (1/2 cup) vegetables preferably broccoli, green beans, mixed vegetables, or salad.
3. (1/2 cup) of fruit. Preferably grapes or orange. You may also have a choice of (1) banana instead of 1/2 cup of fruit.
4. (3) 16 oz bottles or cups of water *(must be completed before bedtime)*

WORKOUT PLAN #1
GOAL: ½ *GALLON OF WATER DAILY*
8 WEEK PROGRAM

********USE THIS WORKOUT PLAN FOR
WEIGHT LOSS ONLY- FOR 8 WEEKS********

Stretching *(do before Walking or Running)*

1. **Hand to toe touches-** (3-sets of 10). *(As you are standing, bend down with legs straight and touch your toes for 10 count. You may do more counts if desire).*
2. **Leg Lunges-** (3-sets of 10) *(leg lunges to the left and to the right).*
3. **Arm Extensions-** *(Pull left and right arm behind your head as you grab your elbow and pull to stretch).*

Walking

1. **WARMUP-** Walk in place or on treadmill for 5 minutes or slowly walk 1 lap around the track, or ½ mile around your neighborhood.
2. **BEGIN FAST PACE WALK WORKOUT-**
   A. Fast Pace Walk 1-3 mile(s) on the treadmill or on the track. *(Length depends on your level. You decrease only as needed.)*
   B. 25 or 50 or 100 jump ropes *(depending on your strength)* (do 3-sets).
3. Repeat stretching to end the day's training.

Running

1. <u>WARMUP-</u> Either run in place or on treadmill for 5 minutes or slowly run 1 lap around the track, or ½ mile around your neighborhood.
2. <u>**BEGIN RUNNING WORKOUT-**</u>
   A. Run 1-3 mile(s) on the treadmill or on the track. *(Length depends on your level.)*
   B. 5- (50) yard sprints.
   C. 25 or 50 or 100 jump ropes *(depending on your strength)*.
3. Repeat stretching to end the day's training.
4. REPEAT training for 5 days each week. SAT and SUN are down (rest) days. NO EXCERSISES should be done during this time. I encourage you to stretch as you rest.

You will repeat this workout for the 8 Week Program none stop. Weigh yourself. You should see immediate results. I have plenty of success stories to prove it.

Lose Weight Fast, Burn Belly Fat Fast in One Day:

(This workout is not added with Workout & Eating Plan #1)
(If you are a beginner, you may do half the workout below).

1. ½ mile run (warm up)
2. 30 high knees (approx. 35-50 yards) (3-5 sets)
3. 60 yard backwards run (3-5 sets)
4. 50-150 jump ropes (depending on your maximum strength) (3-5 sets)
5. 40 yard right and left shuffles (remember to bend your knees as you do each shuffle. (3-5 sets) (depending on your maximum strength)
6. Side hops (1 minute or 30 hops) knees up on each
7. Tuck jumps *with hands straight out* (1 minute or 30 jumps)
8. Mountain Climbers (*sprint up a hill or bleachers and jog back down* -only if you have a hill or bleachers near you) (3-5 sets, your maximum strength desire)
9. ½ mile jogging cool down

You're done for the day. Repeat workout 3-4 times per week. Depending on your maximum workout desire. You may do it 5 times if you have the time and/or in top shape. 2 day rest time.

HINT:
The more you do this workout, the more you will burn fat and calories, the more weight you will lose, and the healthier you will feel. Try doing it straight through for 8-12 weeks for great maximum results.

FYI:
***NO MAXIMUM WORKOUT, NO FAST WEIGHT LOSS RESULTS, OR HEALTHY BODY YOU ARE SHOOTING FOR.

✓ **Obesity Workout & Quick Weight Loss Eating Plan**
Over weight and obesity affects people of all ethnic backgrounds. The best way to illuminate obesity out of your life is through a daily effective and consistent exercise, watching what you eat, controlling the portions of food you put on your plate, and drinking plenty of water daily.

Many children, teens, and adults are suffering with obesity all over the world. Many don't know that they are obese. If you don't know if you are considered obese, below is an example of a person who is 5'9 in height.

Height	Weight Range	Considered
5'9	124 lbs. or less	Underweight
	125 lbs. to 168 lbs.	Heavy weight
	169 lbs. to 202 lbs.	Overweight
	203 lbs. or more	Obese

By studying the chart, the person who is 5'9, which weighs 203 or more pounds is considered obese.

The eating plan and exercises/workout I have provided for you is only an example. You are not obligated to use them if you think they will be harmful to your health or you have not consulted your doctor before attempting them. Please consult your doctor to assure your safety, and so that they will be effective for you.

The Workout (BODY) Plan

Most obesity eating and workout plans take a lot of discipline to do them. However, if you work hard and make them a part of your life, daily, you will see and feel immediate results.

Ready to get started? I know you are. Let's go!

OBESITY EATING PLAN #1
GOAL: 1 *GALLON OF WATER DAILY*
8 WEEK PROGRAM

******USE THIS OBESITY EATING PLAN FOR
QUICK WEIGHT LOSS ONLY- FOR 8 WEEKS******
NOTE: you may drink (8) 16 oz bottled water or drink 1 gallon water daily.

MORNING

1. (3) Egg whites
2. (1) Slice of whole grain toast *(may use low-fat butter)*
3. (1) banana, or apple, or orange
4. (1) Small coffee **-OR-** (1) small juicer/natural fruit drink **-OR-** small protein shake. Drink one in the morning, or noon, or night.
5. (2) 16 oz bottles of water *(must be completed by noon, before lunch)*

**Between breakfast & lunch, you <u>may</u> eat a cup of low-fat jello or low-fat yogurt.

NOON

1. (1 small bowl) of vegetable soup *(no meat), 1/2 cup of fruit* **-OR-**
2. (1) Grilled chicken over a small salad *(low fat dressing)*, (1/2 cup) of fruit. *(Preferably banana, grapes, or orange)*
3. (1) Unsweetened Iced Tea with lemon, **AND** (3) 16 oz bottles of water *(must be completed before dinner)*

**Between lunch & dinner, you <u>may</u> eat a cup of low-fat jello or low-fat yogurt.

71

NIGHT

1. (1) 8 oz baked Fish
2. (1 cup) vegetables *(preferably broccoli, green beans, mixed vegetables)*
3. (1/2 cup) of fruit. Preferably grapes or orange. You may also have a choice of (1) banana instead of 1/2 cup of fruit.
4. (1) Unsweetened Iced Tea with lemon, **AND** (3) 16 oz bottles of water *(must be completed before bedtime)*

OBESITY WORKOUT PLAN #1
GOAL: *½ GALLON OF WATER DAILY*
8 WEEK PROGRAM

******USE THIS WORKOUT PLAN FOR WEIGHT LOSS ONLY- FOR 8 WEEKS******

NOTE: If standing is a strain, or you cannot use your legs, or is 375 pounds or higher, you may have the option to sit while doing these exercises. If you can stand and use your legs, it is recommended.

Stretching *(do before Walking)*

*************STANDING STRETCHES**************

1. **Hand to toe touches-** (3-sets of 10). *(As you are standing, bend down with legs straight and touch your toes for 10 count. You may do more counts if desire).*
2. **Leg Lunges-** (3-sets of 10) *(leg lunges to the left for 10 count and then to the right for 10 count).*
3. **Arm Extensions-** (3-sets of 10) *(Pull left and right arm behind your head as you grab your elbow and pull to stretch for 10 count).*

**************SITTING STRETCHES*****************

1. **Hand to Knee or Calve Touches-** (3-sets of 10). *(As you are sitting, bend down with both hands and touch your knees or calves and back up for 10 count. You may add more counts if desire).*
2. **Sitting Lunges-** (3-sets of 10) *(Hold your right and left arms up and straight out towards your side. You will lean to the left for 10 count, and then to the right for 10 count).*
3. **Arm Extensions-** (3-sets of 10) *(Pull left and right arm behind your head as you grab your elbow and pull to stretch for 10 count each).*
4. **10 Second Arm Rolls-** (3-sets) *(Extend your arms straight out toward your sides and roll them in a forward circular motion as fast as you can for a 10 seconds).*

Walking

**************WALKING IN PLACE***************
***Before beginning, choose whether walking in place or walking is best for you according to what your weight or condition will allow.

1. **WALK IN PLACE WORKOUT-** Walk in place 2-5 minutes, as you move your arms in a running position. Do 5-sets, rest 30 seconds in between each set. *(Once sets are complete, rest for the day, repeat 3-5 days per week)*

******************WALKING*********************

1. **WALK WORKOUT-** Walk 2 laps or 1 mile on the treadmill, or on the track, or at your local park, or around your neighborhood. *(Length depends on your level. You may decrease or increase only as needed.)*
2. Repeat stretches before finishing the day.

IMPORTANT NOTE: You may do 2 days of the Walk in Place Workout <u>or</u> the Walk Workout, and 1 day of the Light Weight Aerobics for a total of a 3-day workout per week. You <u>may</u> increase the more you lose weight and get more in shape. Look below for the Light Weight Aerobics Workout.

Light Weight Aerobics

**************<u>SITTING</u> AEROBICS**************

1. <u>**ARM EXTENTIONS AEROBIC WORKOUT-**</u> With 1 (2-5 pound) dumbbell in <u>each</u> hand, extend your right and left arm out to your side. While keeping your arms straight, lift your arms higher than your head and back down for one count. You will complete 5-10 counts for 3-5 sets. *(**Note:** Please use the dumbbell weight that is suitable for you. Do not increase if it is too heavy. If 2 pounds is too light for you, you may increase to a heavier weight like 3 or 5 pounds or higher.*

2. <u>**ARM EXTENTIONS AEROBIC WORKOUT-**</u> With 1 (2-5 pound) dumbbell in <u>each</u> hand, curl (bring) your dumbbell up to your chest and back down to your side. Complete this at a 5-10 count for 3-5 sets each.

3. <u>**ARM PUNCHING DRILL AEROBIC WORKOUT-**</u> With 1 (2-5 pound) dumbbell in <u>each</u> hand, punch forward and back to your chest. You may alternate punches with your right and left arm, alternating at the same time as you punch right left right left for 5-10 times for 3-5 sets each. *You may increase your count and sets if your level is higher.*

4. <u>**LEG EXTENTIONS AEROBIC WORKOUT-**</u> With 1 (2-5 pound) Leg weight on <u>each</u> leg, alternate your right and left leg as you extend them upward and back down to the floor for 5-10 times for 3-5 sets.

5. <u>**KNEE LIFTS AEROBIC WORKOUT-**</u> With 1 (2-5 pound) Leg weight on <u>each</u> leg, alternate your right and left leg as you lift your knees upward and back down to the floor for 5-10 times for 3-5 sets.

***REPEAT WORKOUTS** for 2-3 days each week. You may do the Light Weight Aerobic workout 1 time added with the Walking Workout only. If you are choosing to <u>only</u> do the Light Weight Aerobic Workout without Walking Workout, you are encouraged to do this exercise 2-3 days per week and increase as you get stronger.

************STANDING AEROBICS*************

1. <u>**ARM EXTENTIONS AEROBIC WORKOUT-**</u> With 1 (2-5 pound) dumbbell in <u>each</u> hand, extend your right and left arm out to your side. While keeping your arms straight, lift your arms higher than your head and back down for one count. You will complete 5-10 counts for 3-5 sets. *(**Note:** Please use the dumbbell weight that is suitable for you. Do not increase if it is too heavy. If 2 pounds is too light for you, you may increase to a heavier weight like 3 or 5 pounds or higher.*

2. <u>**ARM EXTENTIONS AEROBIC WORKOUT-**</u> With 1 (2-5 pound) dumbbell in <u>each</u> hand, curl (bring) your dumbbell up to your chest and back down to your side. Complete this at a 5-10 count for 3-5 sets each.

3. <u>**ARM PUNCHING DRILL AEROBIC WORKOUT-**</u> With 1 (2-5 pound) dumbbell in <u>each</u> hand, punch forward and back to your chest. You may alternate punches with your right and left arm, alternating at the same time as you punch right left right left for 5-10 times for 3-5 sets each. *You may increase your count and sets if your level is higher.*

4. <u>**KICKING LEG EXTENTIONS AEROBIC WORKOUT-**</u> With 1 (2-5 pound) Leg weight on <u>each</u> leg, alternate your right and left leg as you kick outward and back for 5-10 times for 3-5 sets. You may hold 2-5 pound dumbbells in your hand as you kick.

5. <u>**KNEE LIFTS AEROBIC WORKOUT-**</u> With 1 (2-5 pound) Leg weight on <u>each</u> leg, alternate your right and left leg as you lift your knees upward and back down to the floor for 5-10 times for 3-5 sets.

Stephanie Franklin

> **IMPORTANT NOTE:** If weights are too heavy for the Light Weight Aerobic Workout, you may do them without them until you get stronger to use the weight. Using the weights are encouraged. Do your best for best results.

You will repeat this workout(s) for the 8 Week Program none stop. Weigh yourself. You should see immediate results. I have plenty of success stories to prove it. You may repeat the 8 week program as you desire.

PLEASE NOTE:

Above is only 1 sample of my obesity eating plans and exercises/workouts. My more rigorous eating plans and exercises/workouts is made and done in my personal training and boot camp group sessions. To target the eating plan and workout you want, you should contact me for an appointment or workshop, or for a one-day appointment session with you, your group, organization, company, or other to receive a personal training session and a targeting workout to personally fit you.

For more eating plans and a personal workout program that cater to you specifically, please email me at: fitnesshealthbootcamp@gmail.com for a price quote.

If you are interested in making me your personal trainer, please contact me at: fitnesshealthbootcamp@gmail.com.

It does not matter if you live in another town, state, or country, I can still personally train you from where I am located.

I also have additional eating and workout plans for muscle tone, weight gain, toning workouts, Ab workouts for your stomach, agility workouts, strength training workouts, endurance workouts, rehabilitation, and more.

-OR- you may email me to schedule a personal one-on-one personal training and receive your own personal eating plan.

76

Chapter Five

The Spiritual (SOUL) Plan

In thinking of "the Spiritual (SOUL) Plan", one would think in terms of:

❖ **TAKE THE (SOUL) CHALLENGE**

The Spiritual (SOUL) Plan

If you are a believer in God, you will know and realize that you cannot do anything without Him giving you the ability and the strength to do so. We all need God to make it from day to day.

Have you ever met a person who stopped a habit, and weeks later they went back to the same old habit? Well, this happens when a person does not REshape his or herself from the inside out. They are not strong enough on the inside, so their physical body decreases and weakens out. As a result, they return back to the old habits they once changed from. For example, a person starts an 8-week workout and eating program/plan. They quickly lose weight around the second week, and are now disciplined in their eating. Weeks later, a storm comes up in their life and they stress out, give up, and go back to the same old person and/or old habits; and gain the heavy weight back or the sickness comes back. This happened because they did not complete the REshaping process, beginning from the inside out. When you have been REshaped from the inside out, when crises come your way, and because the inner foundation is REshaped, you will be able to endure sudden crises and body fatigue, you will be grounded mentally, and your faith will not fail; but will turn to God for help as you stay motivated and do not quit. You look to God to get stronger.

REshape YOU does surgery on the old person (the way you used to be) on the inside that has a defeated mentality, a faithless walk, and negative attitude about their life. It changes you and opens your eyes to believe that you can make it through every inner storm (obstacle, trial, or challenging situation) that wants you to give up, and turn back to old habits and negative ways of thinking. It also helps you emotionally and through the most stressful times of your life while you're trying to make a turn around by getting yourself together. No one can change you but you. You have to make the decision and stick with it.

As you begin your NEW YOU season, it may be a little stressful as the mind and the body adjusts to the new way of thinking, acting, eating, health wise, and exercising regularly. This is the

The Spiritual (SOUL) Plan

time to allow your Spiritual (SOUL) to kick in and use those scriptures of faith to help you stay determined.

On the next page I challenge you to take the (SOUL) challenge and apply it to your life on a daily basis, as it will help you to grow stronger in your faith to believe that you can be healed from heavy weight, negative let downs, and from believing that you can never make a change to better yourself to the NEW REshaped YOU that you desire to be.

TAKE THE (SOUL) CHALLENGE

Challenge #1
Challenge yourself to go to God when you need help.

Challenge #2
Be persistent and consistent. Do not become weary when you first begin and your body feels tired and it doesn't seem to look better. It may not show on the outside yet, but if you keep going, you will begin to see results.

Challenge #3
Allow God to RE*shape* YOU from the inside out. It may not feel great at first because of the purging, however, as you press your way through, there are great rewards to receive.

Challenge #4
Do not quit. Do not quit. Do not quit. You can do it!

Chapter Six

The Bodybuilding (STRENGTH TRAINNIG) 360 Plan

In thinking of "the Bodybuilding (STRENGTH TRAINING) 360 Plan", one would think in terms of:

- ✓ Low carb workout
- ✓ Consistent protein intake
- ✓ Strength training for endurance
- ✓ Weight training and constant maxing out

The Bodybuilding (STRENGTH TRAINING) 360 Plan

The Bodybuilding (STRENGTH TRAINING) 360 Plan is for the bodybuilder who wants to make a 360 degree turn in your daily diet/eating plan and workout for best results. You have trained and trained and have been unsuccessful in your workouts or in contest(s), and you feel there is still something needed, and you want to win in these areas. This chapter is for you.

There are all sorts of diets/eating plans that help the bodybuilder to get the massive defined muscular body he or she so earnestly desires. Protein intake plays a huge part in the muscular definition. In fact, protein is the breakthrough for the changed muscular body look.

To receive the bodybuilding body you want, it is important to find a plan that works just for you and for your body. Everyone's body structure is different. Muscles define differently on most bodies. Different dietary supplements do not work for everybody as well. In addition, some workouts do not cater to you or to your specific body needs and goals as do others. Therefore, with that said, you have to find the plan that works just for you.

I'll share a true story. There was a time I began back working out after laying off for years. Motivation and preparation was very hard for me. One thing I did not realize was how much fat my body had accumulated over the years and through excessive weight gain. It was very hard for me to lose. I tried working out more and more. I even tried copying others who had a more defined muscular body, and it still did not work. I finally realized that I had to find a eating and workout plan that worked just for me. After finding that eating and workout plan, as I found several, I found that those plans were perfect just for me. So I began to build from there. And, this is what you have got to do, find what works just for you and build from there. Your eating and workout plan may not be like others, but the good news is, is that I am giving you your start and you should be able to build from there and accomplish your goal(s).

✓ **Low Carb workout**

A low carb workout is always the key to winning the results you are looking for with gaining muscle. Although this brings good results, it can also bring soreness, tiredness, and lack of energy as millions of those who have tried this across the world would agree, especially if you're trying the low carb diet. If you are experiencing this, just revamp your exercises and weight lifting to something quick but yet heavy and intense. Quick workout results consume fewer calories than longer workouts. A low carb workout should be implemented to burn fat and increase muscle. This is ideal for the competing bodybuilder.

✓ **Consistent protein intake**

It is important to have the right amount of protein intake. As I have stated before, everybody's body is different whereas some can tolerate more protein than others can, and some do not need excessive amounts.

It depends on the amount of fat you are trying to burn in your body, which will determine how much protein you should intake. However, do not exceed over the right intake.

Read the instructions on the protein container for the right amount and for best results. I have found that taking protein is good with your meal. However, when you take it, it should be consistent and persistent for best results.

✓ **Strength training for endurance**

You want to choose the right strength training for accurate endurance. Much running, jump roping, and rigorous strength trainings are great tools to gain endurance. Most boxers seek after endurance in order to last all of those boxing rounds and constant jabs they endure. However, the bodybuilder is the same but in a different way. He or she need endurance in order to constantly and successfully lift the required heavy weight in competition needed to win the contest. Endurance helps the bodybuilder to last through the most rigorous and tiresome times of training and competitions. If you as a bodybuilder is struggling in this area, below are some bodybuilding (for strength training and defined muscular increase) workouts I'll give you to follow:

1. Medicine Ball Catch and Throw- (need an assistant or trainer). You will catch and throw forward and backwards (throw behind your head). The medicine ball weight should begin no lower than 25 pounds. Higher for maximum weight throw.

2. Plyometric Box or Bench Jumping- (bend your knees as you jump as high as you can over each box or hurdle). You will need a minimum of three boxes (2 ft X 2 ft) or hurdles, and they each should increase in height from the

first box to the third, as you jump over each one without stopping. (5- sets are recommended).

3. Consistent and Persistent heavy weight lifting and knee bending exercises. (5-sets of each recommended).

4. Quick Chest Pushes & Quick Running Release- This is where you will time your pushes in a push-up position for 1 minute to 3-5 minutes, or whatever your max time is. Rapidly push up and down until your max time has expired then quickly thrust up into a fast sprint for 20 to 25 yards to finish. This should be done 3-5 times or as many as your max can go. You can also add weight on your back (10 pounds or higher) to give you more strength and add to more muscular max you are desiring. REMEMBER: Do not overdo it, start where you know you can be consistent and also safe from injury. What may work for another workout friend or someone else, may not work for you yet. Be patient until you get there. This will not be long if it is done right.

As you as a bodybuilder implement these exercises in your trainings, each should increase endurance and strength.

✓ **Weight training and constant maxing out**
As a bodybuilder, weight training and maxing out should be done on a consistent, daily basis. Each day the weights are before you,

you should be experiencing a maxing out experience. I realize some days are for endurance, while others may be for just strength training, and others.

Weight training is very important, and if not done or done properly, you will have negative results. However, if weight training is done properly, with the proper eating plan and rest, you will receive the awards and prestige you are trying to achieve.

Below are a couple of bodybuilding eating plans to get you going. When it comes to finding the right-eating plan for you, there are two diets/eating plans that are essential for you, the body builder.

1. A carb diet/eating plan.
2. A mass gain diet/eating plan.

For the carb diet/eating plan, you can make low-carb mini asparagus and lean turkey bacon muffins, and low-carb stuffed mushroom salad. The ingredients and directions are on next page:

Mini Asparagus & Lean Turkey Bacon Muffins

Ingredients:

- ✓ 1 cup egg beaters
- ✓ 1/2 cup of roasted asparagus
- ✓ 1/2 of chopped extra lean turkey bacon
- ✓ 1/2 tbsp of parsley
- ✓ Muffin mix (no sugar or salt)

Directions:

1. Use a saucepan; add the asparagus and turkey bacon.
2. Stir all together with parsley and eggbeaters.
3. Pour mixture into mini muffin pan and bake at 375 for 8-10 minutes.

NUTRITION FACTS
Calories 196
Total Fat 2g
Total Carb 6g
Protein

Stuffed Mushroom Salad

Ingredients:

- ✓ 1-2 mini bell peppers
- ✓ 1/2 mini heirloom tomatoes
- ✓ 3 oz grilled chicken
- ✓ 2 tbsp Balsamic vinegar
- ✓ 1 low-fat mozzarella cheese either shredded or cut into 1/4 inch slices
- ✓ 1/2 or 1 cup of mushrooms. You may slice as you desire.

✓ Italian seasoning or garlic salt (optional)
✓ 2 tbsp of your choice fat-free, no sugar salad dressing

Directions:

1. Use a large salad bowl.
2. Add and mix salad and all ingredients into large salad bowl.
3. Toss all together with large salad spoons.
4. Serve as desire.

NUTRITION FACTS
SERVING SIZE (1 SALAD)
   Amount per serving
Calories 320
Total Fat10g
Total Carb 31g
Protein 32g
NUTRITION FACTS
STUFFED MUSHROOMS
SERVING SIZE (4 MUSHROOMS)

Amount per serving
Calories 95
Total Fat 1g
Total Carb 6g
Protein 11g

I have provided you with a few bodybuilding strength-training workouts and diet/eating plans just for you. You can add to what I have provided and create more of what may work for you as well.

The Bodybuilding (STRENGTH TRAINING) 360 Plan

Drink plenty of water, protein shakes, protein bars, and nutritious juicing on a daily basis to help lose, and eat away at body fat. Remember to take and eat wisely.

Certainly dietary pill popping may not necessarily get you the lean muscular body you desire. However, a daily and steady well-formatted fat burning workout and tedious healthy eating plan will. It will increase the effects you are looking for and the extra amino in your workout to destroy the war against baby and excessive body fat. Make sense? Good.

You can have the great bodybuilding body you desire if you just:

1. Don't shrug your shoulders and make a bunch of excuses
2. Get going
3. Choose the right bodybuilding <u>workout plan</u> just for you (you may start with the one I gave you)
4. Choose the right bodybuilding <u>eating plan</u> just for you
5. Find the right fat burner just for you
6. Work hard and work up a sweat
7. Be consistent and persistent no matter what, even when you do not get the results you are looking for right away. Be patient, it will come.
8. Motivate and encourage others

As you take this challenge offered in this chapter to get the bodybuilding and strength-training body you desire, you will make a complete 360 degree turn around in your weightlifting, strength-training workouts, the massive muscular body you want, and the healthy living to round it all off cohesively together.

Chapter Seven

Experience the NEW RE*shaped* YOU

Are you ready to be REshaped? Have you gone through each chapter and the process in this book to experience the NEW REshaped YOU? I can tell you it feels great to experience the NEW REshaped YOU. The only example I can give is when you first step out of a hot bubble bath, the cleansing you feel after you wash off the old dirt and grim from the stress of the day, and put on the NEW REshaped YOU, a clean NEW look, which is actually far better than what the example can give.

You no longer feel heavy and bound. You feel light and a NEW YOU. This is what I mean by experiencing the NEW REshaped YOU. I encourage you to experience it today!

On the next page, I have given you some detailed eating plan suggestions as you experience the NEW REshaped YOU.

Weight Loss Eating Plan Suggestion:
You may ask the question, "how much should I weigh?" I will answer, with a proper eating plan, you should weigh the proper weight for your height.

With a weight loss diet/eating plan, you can lower your blood pressure, blood sugar (diabetes), and risk of heart decease.

Here is a Weight Loss Eating Plan Suggestion Below:
Stay away from breads as much as possible (wheat breads recommended only if eating bread).

Weight loss can come through a low-carbohydrate diet/eating plan. This can prevent many health conditions and issues. If followed, it can reduce the risk of health issues.

Here's How it Works:
Low-Carbohydrate Diet below-
- Protein
- Vegetables
- Healthy fat

Whole Grains-
- Barley
- Oaks
- Rice *(brown rice)*

Forbidden Foods You Should Not Eat-
- White sugar
- White rice
- White bread
- White potatoes

- Pasta made with flour
- Starchy vegetables
- Dairy products
- Alcohol

Your goal should be to rev up your body's ability to burn fat. As you lose the weight you can add some carbohydrates back into your diet/eating plan such as:

- Berries
- Yogurt
- Nuts
- Fruits

Your goal should be to stick to the diet/eating plan and lose until you are at your desired weight.

Chapter Bonus!

Diabetic Eating Plan & Workout

- ✓ Eating plan
- ✓ The bottom line
- ✓ Burning fat: *Daily workout*
- ❖ **TAKE THE WORKOUT CHALLENGE**

Diabetes is one of the number one killers in the world and can shorten a person's life. Believe it or not, enormous weight gain and poor eating habits are mostly the hindering problem. How you help eliminate this terrible sickness is by constantly working out and eating a healthy balanced diet/eating plan.

Although there are many different eating plans and workout programs, there are not many that cater to diabetics. There are many different reasons to exercise, as weight loss may not be the center focus. You may do simple exercises that can improve your balance, flexibility, energy level, and feeling of well-being, which makes accomplishing these tasks within your daily life much more easier.

Not dealing with poor eating habits is the world's obsession. Not focusing on good eating habits are the world's biggest let down. As these have been a power outage to many and have caused great grief, insecurity, and let downs, there have been changes many have made and are determined to change. If you notice, the world is much more focused on eating and exercising better with all the fitness programs offered everywhere. There are more dietary (eating plans) solutions offered whether on television or all over the internet. There is also a lot of fitness DVD's, workouts, and books that offer the best solution to getting a great healthy and fit body.

Just because you are a diabetic, does not mean it is the end of the world. I have family members that are diabetics and they are coping as normal individuals that have decided to make proper changes to workout, and to their diets and eating habits. As they have made the change, they have been successful and you can too.

✓ **Eating Plan**

Practically the entire world is concerned about losing weight. No one wants to gain weight and have to deal with being overweight. As one intake fatty meals, the body increases fatty tissues. Fatty acids absorb and transport to the liver, where essential nutrients are removed. The rest are packaged together with proteins to form chylomicrons, so that it can travel throughout the bloodstream to all the organs and cells that need it. This is why it is important not to eat fatty foods. If you eat more fat than the body needs, it either gets stored in the arteries of your heart—which is not a good thing, or it can also can get stored in your liver—which can give you a fatty liver, and can spread to your hips, thighs, buttocks, or abdomen; which is also not a good thing.

✓ **The Bottom Line**
The bottom line is, we are all in this together, and we all need each other. It is very important to live a healthy life with healthy eating habits and a daily healthy workout plan. There are so many out there that you really don't know which ones to join or become a part of. The best result is to find what plan works for you and which one you feel comfortable with as I have stated before in the book. Everyone is different, and every person's body is not the same. This is why you should look for the right eating plan that works just for you, and a consistent workout plan that you know you are going to start good, and be consistent to complete each day of your life as I have also stated throughout the book.

✓ Burning Fat: *Daily Workout*

There are vital keys to burning fat. Two of which are running and weight lifting. These two coincide together. They both work side by side as they both agree with burning fat in the body.

Your muscles burn calories and help you maintain your metabolic rate. The more fat you burn, the more muscle you gain. The more muscle you gain, the more lean your body will be and the healthier you will look and feel.

If you are a diabetic and/or diabetes run in your family, it is recommended that you take your workouts and eating plans more seriously. The more you workout, the more you will lose weight and the less chance you will have to inherit diabetes. While no one can say if a person workout, they will not receive diabetes. However, you want to take as much precaution as possible. I have seen in people I know who had type 1 diabetes do these things—workout on a daily basis and follow a healthy eating plan, get healed from this sickness. They went from taking insulin 4 times per day, to no insulin or pills at all.

A consistent and persistent, daily workout while sticking to a healthy diet/eating plan, will increase your chances of being healed from diabetes.

A good nutritious eating plan is a great thing to burn fat and have a healthy, great fit body. I have an example for you. The more green foods (green beans, spinach, cabbage, celery, and salads), the better you will feel. When I first started changing my eating plan to a more healthy eating plan, I must admit it was a challenge at first, and at times it still is. However, once you continue on it and do not give up as you make it a way of life, it will become easier for you. My mother struggled with type 1 diabetes for over thirty years and changing from eating fatty foods, fried foods, regular take-outs, sodas, and foods that have sugar in them, was very hard for her. However, as I pushed and motivated her, she made up in her mind that she was going to change. She knew that her health depended on her change, she took each day as is, started walking and changed from all the fatty foods, fried foods, replaced the sodas with much water and sugar free drinks; and foods without sugar added, brought her weight down quickly and tremendously; and her sugar level went down also. So, it works, but you have to have a made up mind and determination that you are going to change and get yourself together. You are not defeated. You can win just as she did and be determined as she is. I encourage you to live a gluten-free, fatty free, and sugar free lifestyle!

BEFORE STARTING THE EXERCISES

Due to conditions such as high blood pressure and certain diabetes, complication can make certain activities less safe. You should, as with diabetes, be advised to see a doctor for a checkup before starting these exercises below.

Once you get the approval or have already, then let's begin. The workout and eating plan will provide guidance on how to complete them and complete them safely.

YOUR GOAL SHOULD BE BEFORE BEGINNING:

FROM YOUR MEALS- Remove fat, remove sugar, lower sodium, reduce portions (amounts per meal), and add fiber. Sweets and fatty foods can be challenging. However, take one day at a time as you use other replacements to accomplish this plan successfully.

When preparing meals with meat and poultry, lower the fat, saturated fat, and cholesterol in your meal by replacing them with lean cuts of meat, take the skin off poultry, and reduce that amount of meat in your eating plan and recipe. For example, make smaller hamburgers, or use ¾ of a pound of ground turkey breast meat, or 95% lean ground beef instead. Chicken and turkey are good meats to add to your diet/eating plan.

Foods that are high in saturated fat include fatty red meats, butter, cheese, cream, whole milk, and coconut oil. Foods that are high in *trans*-fat include margarines and shortening. Other sources of *trans*-fat include many commercially baked goods, such as crackers with salt, cookies, and cakes, and commercially fried foods, such as, french fries and donuts. When shopping for your meals, try replacing the butter, margarine that contains *trans*-fat, shortenings with liquid vegetable oils such as canola oils, flaxseed, peanut, olive, safflower, or sunflower oils.

Sugar substitutes can be used to replace sugar in some items. Foods that rely on sugar for their structure, such as cakes, cookies, muffins, and quick breads, you should replace them with low-calorie sweeteners. For foods in which sugar is used primarily for its sweet taste, such as beverages (sodas), sauces, marinades, frozen desserts, puddings, custards, and fruit fillings for pies and cobblers, you may be able to replace all of the sugar with low-calorie sweeteners.

Most sodium foods that have salt or high-sodium ingredients added during processing or preparation usually are high in sodium. To eliminate this, you can prepare your foods with herbs, spices, or garlic to compensate for less salt. You can also seek out low-sodium or reduced-sodium ingredients when cooking broth, canned or dried soups, or canned vegetables. In some of your dishes, you may be able to substitute fresh ingredients, such as, fresh tomatoes in place of canned.

Fiber is an essential part of a healthy diet and eating plan. It helps lower blood glucose, blood cholesterol, and blood pressure levels. It also helps to maintain a healthy colon and promotes weight control since high-fiber foods causes you to feel fuller with fewer calories.

Stephanie Franklin

Holiday seasons are the worst when trying to lower portion sizes in your dishes. There are ways to avoid over eating such dishes when you make them regularly, whether during holiday seasons or not. One perfect way is to reduce your portion amount. If you currently add 1 cup of each serving to your plate, you would want to reduce them by ½ each serving. This can successfully be done by using measuring cups until you are confident in knowing how much to serve yourself per plate. I have tried this and it has been successfully rewarding. By lowering your portion amounts per dish, can quickly lower your weight and gluten desire.

I want to show you an example you may want to follow for yourself and family below of how your plate should look each time you eat. Most people think that meat should be the largest portion on the plate. However, it's not, it should be the same portion of the starches, as the vegetables should be the largest portion served. Look at the diagram below.

How your dinner plate should look

Starches | Meats

Vegetables

On the next page begins the eating and workout plan I have provided for you to follow to complete. I only share one of each as they can help give you a start and a daily guide to a healthy successful workout and eating plan. You can add to it or put your own together now that you see how to do it and what new choices I give you.

DIABETIC EATING PLAN #1
GOAL: ½ *GALLON OF WATER DAILY*
Try for 8 WEEKS and After PROGRAM

******USE THIS EATING PLAN FOR QUICK WEIGHT LOSS ONLY- FOR 8 WEEKS******

ONE STEP AT A TIME: Remove fat, remove sugar, lower sodium, reduce portions (amounts per meal), and add fiber.

MORNING
1. (1) EGG
2. (1) SLICE OF TOAST *(wheat bread, -OR- whole wheat bagel (1 ½ ounces).*
3. 1/2 cup of oatmeal *(quick oats- not instant oats)*
4. For a rushed morning, you may eat cereal that has fiber and no sugar added.
5. (1) juicer/natural fruit drink. *Drink one in the morning, or noon, or night.*
6. (2) 16 oz bottles or cups of water *(must be completed by noon, before lunch).* You may also drink skim milk *(optional).*

NOON
1. (1) Sandwich *(wheat bread only with turkey or ham).*
2. (1) bag of chips preferably "All Natural Chips or Tortilla Chips"*(no salt).*
3. **-OR-** instead of sandwich and chips, you may do (1 cup) of vegetable soup (unsalted less meat). And saltine crackers *(optional)*
4. (1 cup) of fruit. *Preferably grapes or orange.*
5. (3) 16 oz bottles or cups of water *(must be completed before dinner)*

NIGHT

1. (1 slice) Baked chicken or turkey
2. (1/2 cup) vegetables *(preferably broccoli, green beans, mixed vegetables).*
3. (1/2 cup) of salad *(spinach, pineapple, cucumber, or tuna, or your choice).*
4. (1/2 cup) of fruit. Preferably grapes or orange. *(You may also have a choice of (1) banana instead of 1/2 cup of fruit).*
5. (3) 16 oz bottles or cups of water *(must be completed before bedtime)*

DIABETIC WORKOUT PLAN #1
GOAL: ½ *GALLON OF WATER DAILY*
Try for 8 WEEKS and After PROGRAM

******USE THIS WORKOUT PLAN FOR WEIGHT LOSS ONLY- FOR 8 WEEKS******

Stretching *(do before Walking or Running)*

1. **Hand to toe touches-** (3-sets of 10). *(As you are standing, bend down with legs straight and touch your toes for 10 count. You may do more counts if desire).*
2. **Leg Lunges-** (3-sets of 10) *(leg lunges to the left and to the right).*
3. **Arm Extensions-** (3-sets of 10) *(Pull left and right arm behind your head as you grab your elbow and pull to stretch).*

Walking *(you may walk or run, or do both)*

1. <u>WARM UP-</u> Walk slowly in place or on a treadmill for 5 minutes, or slowly walk 1 lap around the track, or around your neighborhood.
2. <u>BEGIN WALK WORKOUT-</u>
   A. Walk 1-3 mile(s) on the treadmill or on the track. *(Length depends on your level. You may decrease only as needed.)*
   B. 25 or 50 or 100 jump ropes *(depending on your strength)* (do 3-sets).
   C. 25 ft. Lunges. *(turn to right side and lung for 25ft. going, left side coming back)*
   D. 25 ft. Knee Highs. *(Knee high for 25 ft. and back)*
   E. Repeat stretching to end the day's workout.

PLEASE NOTE: If exercises are too rigorous with your condition, you may only walk slow until you gain your strength to increase to the exercises.

Running *(you may walk or run, or do both)*

1. <u>WARM UP-</u> Either, run in place **or,** on a treadmill for 5 minutes **or,** slowly trot 1 lap around the track, **or,** ½ mile around your neighborhood.
2. <u>**BEGIN RUNNING WORKOUT-**</u>
   A. Run 1-3 mile(s) on the treadmill or on the track *(Length depends on your level).*
   B. 25 or, 50 or, 100 jump ropes *(depending on your strength).*
   C. Repeat stretching to end the day's training.
   D. REPEAT training for 5 days each week. SAT and SUN are down (rest) days. NO EXCERSISES should be done during this time. I encourage you to stretch as you rest and drink plenty of water.

<u>*PLEASE NOTE:*</u> If exercises are too rigorous with your condition, you may only walk slowly until you gain your strength to increase to the exercises.

Weight Lifting

1. **Leg Lifts-** Use 3-5 pound ankle weights. Lay down on right side, while keeping your leg straight, and lift leg 10-20 times or to your maximum count. Turn and repeat left side. *(If ankle weights are too heavy, you may do exercise without them) (Repeat 3 sets).*
2. **10-25, 50-100 Sit-Ups-** *(You may increase your count to your maximum count).*
3. **Arm Curls-** Use (2) 2 pound or your maximum hand held dumbbells. *(With dumbbells in each hand, curl your hand held dumbbells up to your shoulders and back down for 10-15 times, or your maximum count. You may do both arms at the same time or you may do them one at a time) (Do 3-sets of 10-15 arm curls).*

4. **Arm Lifts-** Use (2) 2 pound or your maximum hand held dumbbell. *(With dumbbells in each hand, while keeping your arms straight, lift dumbbell up higher than your head, and back down to your legs. Do 3-sets of 10-15 arm curls or your maximum count).*

***You will repeat this Diabetic Workout Plan for the 8 Week Program, none stop. After program, you may repeat if desire. You should see immediate results. I have plenty of success stories to prove it.

TAKE THE DIABETIC CHALLENGE

Challenge #1
Challenge yourself to eat healthy.

Challenge #2
Be persistent and consistent in working out. Do not become weary when you first begin and your body feels tired and it doesn't seem to look better. It may not show on the outside yet, but if you keep going, you will begin to see results in your health and in your body.

Challenge #3
Exercise everyday and have faith in yourself.

Challenge #4
Experience the **Re*shaped* NEW YOU** from the inside out.

You can accomplish these exercises from home, a local park, gym, and can be done with a workout partner, group, and/or alone.

Conclusion

While no one's perfect and we all are trying to get where we all need to be, I encourage you to raise the standard within yourself by holding yourself accountable for your health and weight. Run toward the mark to RE*shape* the **NEW YOU**. You will not only feel great, but you will also look great with a completely new determination on the inside and a NEW outlook on life and your future on the outside.

The RE*shape* YOU Workbook

Set Your Goals

Joint Down Completed Goals

What Diets/Eating plans have you Started?

What Diets/Eating plans have you completed?

Note Pad

Stephanie Franklin

Note Pad

Stephanie Franklin

1. **Chapter Two:** page 35, *"a mind is a terrible thing to waste"*
(http://en.wikipedia.org/wiki/United_Negro_College_Fund)

(http://www.adcouncil.org/Our-Campaigns/The-Classics/United-Negro-College-Fund)

A mind is a terrible thing to waste.
(http://www.answers.com/Q/What_is_the_origin_of_the_phrase_'A_mind_is_a_terrible_thing_to_waste')

2. **Chapter Bonus:** American Diabetes Association-
(http://www.diabetes.org/?loc=logo)

3. **Chapter Four:** The Weight of the Nation
(http://theweightofthenation.hbo.com)

Height chart-
(http://theweightofthenation.hbo.com/themes/what-is-obesity)

4. Scripture quotations are from the Holy Bible. *Zondervan, 1995. Grand Rapids, Michigan.*

Contact Me

Stephanie is a personal trainer, coach, counselor, and motivational speaker. For more information and bookings, and if you would like her to be your Personal Trainer, and/or sign up for her Fitness & Health (group) Boot Camp Program, please email her at:

fitnesshealthbootcamp@gmail.com

In your email, please make sure to add your name, phone, email, and what type of service you would like:

1. Personal Training
2. Fitness Health (group) Boot Camp Program

**Without this information, Stephanie will not be able to return your email.

MEET THE AUTHOR

Stephanie is using her years of credentials and personal experiences as a personal trainer and coach to share through her life-changing book, "REshape YOU", which comes to change the heart, mind, body, and soul from the inside out. She is excited about what it is already accomplishing in the lives of athletes, leaders, church ministries, youth, those struggling with obesity, and people who just want to win in lowering their weight, their fitness needs, health needs, and entire being.

www.ingramcontent.com/pod-product-compliance
Lightning Source LLC
Chambersburg PA
CBHW071229290326
41931CB00037B/2536